VALUE GUIDE'S FORAGING FOR HERABL REMEDIES

T. Pilinski

Blurb

"Value Guide's Foraging Herbal Remedies" is your concise companion on the journey to understanding and utilizing the healing powers of nature. This guide unlocks the secrets of several common and easily found potent herbs—from the liver-cleansing milk thistle to the soothing chamomile and invigorating peppermint—providing you with the knowledge to identify, harvest, and harness their medicinal qualities.

Crafted for nature enthusiasts, herbalists, and anyone interested in alternative health, this book blends scientific insights with traditional wisdom to offer practical, hands-on advice, ensuring you can safely and sustainably explore the benefits of natural remedies. Whether you're a novice forager or an experienced herbalist, this guide will enrich your understanding of herbal medicine and inspire a deeper connection with the world around you. Embark on this enlightening path to discover the scientific underpinnings and therapeutic benefits of herbs, enriching your health and deepening your connection with nature.

Introduction

Welcome to "Value Guide's Foraging Herbal Remedies," a comprehensive Value Guide meticulously crafted for nature enthusiasts, herbalists, and anyone curious about the manifold health benefits our natural surroundings offer. As you turn these pages, you'll embark on a transformative journey through the wilds of your backyard, the hidden nooks of local parks, and the pristine expanses of untouched natural landscapes. Here, you'll uncover a world of herbs that not only heal and soothe but also deeply nourish the body and soul.

In recent years, we've observed a significant resurgence in holistic health practices, a revival characterized by a growing disillusionment with conventional pharmaceuticals and a renewed interest in natural remedies. This guide is a direct response to that paradigm shift, offering practical knowledge and hands-on advice for safely harnessing nature's bounty. With an increasing number of people striving to reduce their chemical load and reconnect with the earth, herbal remedies provide a timely and enduring solution rooted in age-old wisdom and practice.

Our goal extends beyond mere education. We aim to transform how you interact with the natural world. Each chapter of this guide delves into one of eleven common yet potent herbs, detailing their medicinal properties, methods of identification and harvest, and their culinary potentials. From the liver-cleansing power of milk thistle to the calming effects of chamomile, these herbs are not merely accessible but are indispensable for a well-rounded approach to health and well-being.

It is essential to note that while herbal remedies can offer significant health benefits, they are not a substitute for professional medical advice. Always consult with a healthcare provider before starting any new treatment, especially if you have existing health conditions or are taking other medications. This book is designed to enlighten and inspire, equipped with the caution and respect these powerful plants demand.

Let's step into the green, armed with knowledge and a spirit of adventure, ready to explore the healing power of plants. This journey promises not only to enhance your understanding of herbal medicine but also to deepen your connection with the environment. It will foster a greater appreciation for the plants that thrive around us and teach us how to live in harmony with our surroundings.

Whether you are a seasoned herbalist or a novice forager, "Foraging Herbal Remedies" will open your eyes to the wonders of the natural pharmacy that grows just beyond your doorstep. You will learn how to prepare remedies that soothe, invigorate, and heal; how to blend science with tradition in your herbal practice; and how to cultivate a lifestyle that embraces the holistic values of sustainability, wellness, and balance.

Prepare to be transformed by the knowledge and beauty of the natural world as we embark on this green path together, discovering the profound healing power that lies in the simple act of connecting with the earth. Welcome to your herbal adventure.

Ready to embrace the wisdom of the wild? As you learn to identify, harvest, and utilize these herbs, you'll gain more than just an understanding of their uses. You'll develop a deeper connection with the environment. This guide aims to foster a sustainable foraging practice that respects the ecosystems from which we draw these resources.

Throughout this book, you'll find detailed descriptions of each herb's appearance, the best times and places for harvesting, and how to prepare them for both medicinal and culinary uses. We'll explore the specific health benefits of each herb, supported by both traditional uses and modern research, to provide you with the most comprehensive and actionable information possible.

Remember, foraging isn't just about taking. It's about giving back. We'll discuss the ethics of sustainable foraging and how to harvest responsibly so these plants can continue to thrive in their natural habitats for generations to come.

As you turn each page, imagine the crunch of leaves underfoot, the fresh scent of soil, and the thrill of finding your first sprig of wild peppermint or dandelion root. This book isn't just a guide. It's an invitation to adventure and a call to explore the untamed parts of the world.

As we move forward, consider this book not only a tool but also a companion on your foraging journeys. Each chapter has been meticulously designed to guide you safely and effectively. You'll learn how to spot these herbs with ease, understand their life cycles, and harness their natural properties for your use.

This guide also serves as a bridge between ancient wisdom and contemporary science, offering a balanced perspective that respects both the old and new schools of thought in the realm of natural medicine. Whether you're a novice to the world of herbal remedies or an experienced forager, there's something in these pages for everyone.

By the end of this book, you will not only be proficient in identifying and using these remarkable herbs, but you will also be inspired to continue your exploration of herbal medicine. Perhaps you'll feel compelled to grow some of these herbs in your own garden, share your knowledge with friends, or even advocate for the preservation of natural spaces where these plants thrive.

Thank you for choosing to embark on this green path with "Foraging Herbal Remedies." Here's to your health, happiness, and the countless adventures that await in the great outdoors. So, lace up your boots, grab your basket, and let's begin this journey together. With "Foraging Herbal Remedies" in hand, you're not just a reader. You're an explorer, poised on the brink of countless green discoveries. Let's get foraging!

Chapter 1: The Rise of Holistic Health

In recent years, there has been a noticeable shift back toward holistic health—a movement that embraces the totality of individuals, including their physical, mental, emotional, and environmental well-being. This chapter delves into why holistic approaches, particularly those involving herbal remedies and foraging, are not only gaining popularity but are also essential in today's health landscape.

1.1 Understanding Holistic Health

Holistic health is founded on the principle that each aspect of a person's life contributes to their overall health. Unlike traditional medicine, which often focuses on treating specific ailments, holistic practices aim to bring balance to the entire body and mind. This comprehensive approach can include diet, exercise, mental health care, and, of course, the use of natural remedies.

1.2 History and Resurgence

For centuries, herbal medicine was the cornerstone of healthcare. Ancient texts and archaeological findings from various cultures show the extensive use of plants for medicinal purposes. However, with the rise of pharmaceuticals, these natural methods were overshadowed. Now, we're witnessing a resurgence of interest in these ancient practices as people seek safer, more sustainable, and less invasive ways to manage their health.

1.3 Scientific Support for Herbal Remedies

Recent studies have begun to validate what traditional herbalists have known for generations—plants possess potent medicinal properties that can support health in many ways. From the anti-inflammatory effects of nettles to the liver-protecting properties of milk thistle, science is starting to acknowledge the value of these natural remedies.

1.4 Modern Adoption and Popularity

The integration of holistic health into mainstream culture is evident from the growth of organic food sales, the popularity of yoga and meditation, and the increasing use of herbal supplements. More healthcare practitioners are now recommending herbal remedies as complementary therapies, illustrating a broader acceptance of their benefits.

1.5 Addressing the Skeptics

Despite growing evidence and popularity, holistic medicine still faces skepticism. Critics often cite a lack of rigorous scientific research or regulatory oversight as major concerns. However, many herbal remedies have a long history of safe use, supported by emerging research and a better understanding of their mechanisms.

1.6 The Importance of Being Informed

As with any approach to health, being well-informed is crucial. This means understanding not only the benefits but also the limitations and potential risks of herbal remedies. It's important to consult healthcare providers, especially when considering herbs for serious or chronic conditions.

This chapter sets the stage for the rest of the book by providing a solid foundation in the principles of holistic health and herbal medicine. As we move forward, we'll explore how you can safely and effectively incorporate these ancient practices into your modern lifestyle, starting with the fundamentals of foraging in the next chapter.

Chapter 2: Foraging Fundamentals

Foraging for herbs is both an art and a science. It requires knowledge, respect for nature, and a keen eye. This chapter introduces the essentials of foraging, focusing on how to safely and sustainably collect herbs from the wild. By understanding these fundamentals, you can ensure that your foraging efforts are both productive and environmentally conscious.

2.1 Getting Started with Foraging

Before you begin foraging, it's important to equip yourself with the right tools and knowledge. A good field guide specific to your region, a pair of gardening gloves, scissors or pruning shears, and a basket or bag for your finds are essential. Additionally, understanding the laws and regulations regarding foraging in your area is crucial to ensure that you're collecting legally and ethically.

2.2 Best Practices for Safe Foraging

Safety is paramount when foraging for herbs. Always:

- **Identify plants accurately**: Mistaking one plant for another can be dangerous. Double-check your identifications with a reliable guide or app.

- **Be aware of your surroundings**: Foraging in unfamiliar areas can lead to accidents. Be mindful of the terrain and wildlife.

- **Avoid contaminated areas**: Avoid plants from roadsides, industrial areas, or places that might be sprayed with pesticides or herbicides.

2.3 Ethical Foraging

Sustainable foraging ensures that plants and their habitats remain healthy and viable for future generations. Follow these guidelines:

- **Take only what you need**: Never overharvest. A good rule is to take no more than one-third of the available plants in any given area.

- **Leave no trace**: Be mindful of the environment. Avoid trampling other plants and disturbing wildlife.

- **Spread seeds**: If possible, help the plants reproduce by spreading seeds as you forage.

2.4 Timing and Techniques

Understanding the best time to forage for specific herbs is crucial for maximizing their medicinal and nutritional properties. For example, many roots are best harvested in early spring or late fall when plants store nutrients in their roots. Leaves and flowers, however, should be collected when the plants are in full bloom for the highest potency.

2.5 Processing Your Harvest

Once you've gathered your herbs, proper cleaning, drying, or preparation is key to preserving their beneficial properties. Proper preparation and storage are crucial to maintaining the potency and effectiveness of herbal remedies. Here are some fundamental techniques to ensure the longevity and efficacy of your herbs:

- **Cleaning**: Start by gently washing your herbs under cool running water to remove any dirt, insects, or contaminants. This ensures that the herbs are clean and safe for use in any preparations.

- **Drying**: Properly drying herbs is essential to preserve their medicinal properties.

    - **Air Drying**: Tie the herbs in small bunches and hang them upside down in a warm, dry, and well-ventilated area out of direct sunlight.

o **Oven Drying**: Spread herbs on a baking sheet and place them in an oven set to the lowest temperature. Keep the door slightly open to allow moisture to escape.

o **Using a Dehydrator**: For a more

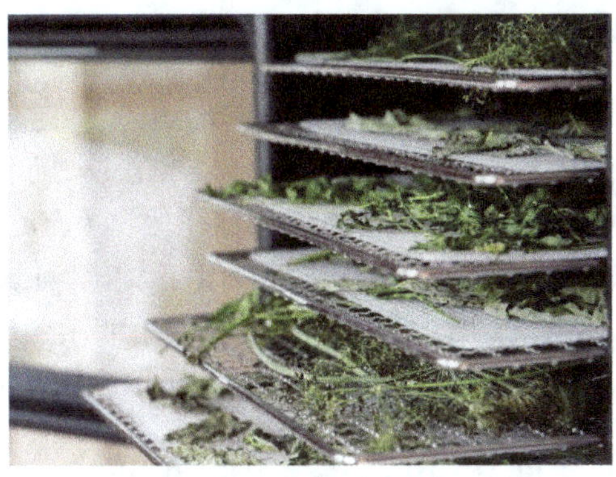

Dehydrator With Herbs.

uniform and efficient drying process, use a dehydrator, following the manufacturer's instructions regarding temperature and duration.

- **Storage**: Storing herbs correctly is critical to retain their therapeutic benefits.

  o **Containers**: Use airtight containers, preferably made of glass, to prevent exposure to air and moisture.

  o **Environment**: Store the containers in a cool, dark place to protect the herbs from light and heat, which can degrade their active compounds.

By implementing these techniques, you can ensure that your herbal remedies remain effective and potent, providing the maximum health benefits whenever you need them.

2.6 Local Laws and Foraging Rights

Foraging isn't free-for-all. It's governed by specific regulations that vary by location. This part of the chapter will provide a general overview of how to find out about foraging laws in your area and the importance of adhering to these rules to promote responsible foraging practices.

By mastering these foraging fundamentals, you'll be ready to explore the specific herbs detailed in the following chapters. Each herb offers unique benefits and challenges, and understanding how to approach foraging with respect and knowledge will enhance your ability to use these natural gifts effectively and sustainably.

Chapter 3: Overview of Featured Herbs

This chapter serves as an introduction to the ten herbs we'll explore in detail throughout this book. Each herb has been chosen not only for its medicinal benefits but also for its accessibility to beginner foragers. Here, we provide a brief overview of each herb, setting the stage for the more comprehensive discussions that follow in later chapters.

3.1 Milk Thistle (Silybum marianum)

- **Medicinal Properties**: Known for its liver-protective qualities, milk thistle is often used to detoxify and repair liver damage.

- **Identifying Features**: Look for shiny, pale green leaves with white veins and large, purple flower heads.

- **Best Seasons to Forage**: Early spring for young leaves, and late summer for seeds.

3.2 Dandelion Root (Taraxacum officinale)

- **Medicinal Properties**: A powerhouse for digestion and skin health, dandelion root is also a natural diuretic.

- **Identifying Features**: Bright yellow flowers and deeply toothed, lance-shaped leaves.

- **Best Seasons to Forage**: Spring and fall for roots; flowers and leaves in spring.

3.3 Plantain (Plantago major)

- **Medicinal Properties**: Offers natural pain relief and is useful in treating wounds and respiratory issues.

- **Identifying Features**: Broad, oval leaves with parallel veins.

- **Best Seasons to Forage**: Spring and early summer when the leaves are most tender.

3.4 Wild Lettuce (Lactuca virosa)

- **Medicinal Properties**: Known for its sedative and pain-relieving properties, useful in managing mild pain and promoting sleep.

- **Identifying Features**: Tall, leafy stems with small yellow buds and milky sap.

- **Best Seasons to Forage**: Late spring through early summer when the leaves are tender and before the sap becomes too bitter.

3.5 Nettles (Urtica dioica)

- **Medicinal Properties**: Rich in nutrients, nettles are used for allergy relief and are known for their anti-inflammatory properties.

- **Identifying Features**: Heart-shaped leaves with a serrated edge and fine hairs that sting on touch.

- **Best Seasons to Forage**: Early spring when the young shoots are most tender.

3.6 Chamomile (Matricaria chamomilla)

- **Medicinal Properties**: Widely used for its calming effects, helpful in treating insomnia and digestive issues.

- **Identifying Features**: Small, daisy-like flowers with a sweet, apple-like fragrance.

- **Best Seasons to Forage**: Late spring to early summer when flowers are in bloom.

3.7 Elderberry (Sambucus nigra)

- **Medicinal Properties**: Immune-boosting capabilities, particularly effective in treating colds and flu.

- **Identifying Features**: Clusters of tiny, white or cream flowers followed by dark purple berries.

- **Best Seasons to Forage**: Summer for flowers, early fall for ripe berries.

3.8 Yarrow (Achillea millefolium)

- **Medicinal Properties**: Used for its wound-healing abilities and for reducing fever.

- **Identifying Features**: Feathery foliage and clusters of small, white to pink flowers.

- **Best Seasons to Forage**: Late spring and summer when in full bloom.

3.9 Burdock (Arctium lappa)

- **Medicinal Properties**: Known to purify blood and support lymphatic drainage.

- **Identifying Features**: Large, broad leaves and prickly seed heads that stick to clothing.

- **Best Seasons to Forage**: Late fall for roots and seeds and leaves throughout the growing season.

3.10 Lemon Balm (Melissa officinalis)

- **Medicinal Properties**: Effective in relieving stress and anxiety, with a mild sedative effect.

- **Identifying Features**: Light green leaves with a lemon scent when crushed.

- **Best Seasons to Forage**: Late spring through early fall.

3.11 Peppermint (Mentha piperita)

- **Medicinal Properties**: Excellent for digestive health, also used to relieve headaches and clear sinus congestion.

- **Identifying Features**: Dark green, serrated leaves with a distinctive minty aroma.

- **Best Seasons to Forage**: Spring and summer for the most potent flavor and medicinal benefits.

With these herbs, you'll have a diverse palette of natural remedies at your fingertips. Each chapter that follows will dive deeper into how to forage, prepare, and use these herbs in various applications, ensuring you can harness their full potential safely and effectively. Let's continue our journey into the green world, one herb at a time.

Chapter 4: Milk Thistle

Milk thistle is not only a striking plant visually but also a powerhouse of medicinal benefits, particularly known for its supportive role in liver health. This chapter explores the plant in depth, emphasizing the active compounds responsible for its benefits.

4.1 Medicinal Properties

- **Liver Protection and Detoxification**: Milk thistle's primary active ingredient, silymarin, a group of compounds including silibinin, silidianin, and silicristin, is celebrated for its liver-protective qualities. Silymarin acts as a potent antioxidant, scavenging harmful free radicals produced by metabolizing toxic substances like alcohol and certain medications. According to research published in the *World Journal of Hepatology*, silymarin enhances hepatic glutathione, boosting the liver's antioxidant capacity, and may also enhance protein synthesis in liver cells, promoting liver tissue regeneration (Vargas-Mendoza et al., 2014).

- **Anti-inflammatory and Antiviral Properties**: Silymarin's anti-inflammatory properties aid in reducing liver inflammation. The same study suggests silymarin has antiviral capabilities that can inhibit the entry of viruses into liver cells, offering potential benefits in treating viral hepatitis.

4.2 Identifying Milk Thistle

- **Appearance**: Recognizable by its glossy,

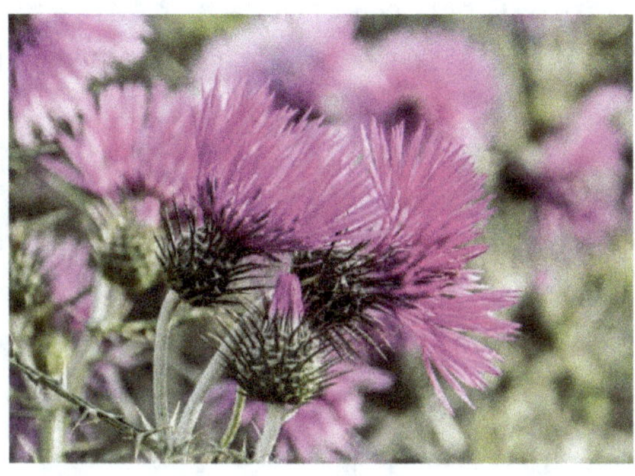

lobed leaves with distinct white veins and purple to reddish-pink thistle-like flowers, milk

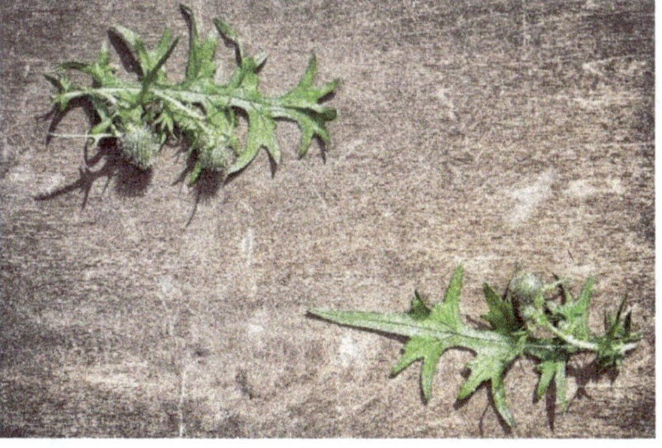

thistle is not only medicinal but also ornamental.

- **Habitat**: Thriving in dry, rocky soils, it is often found in waste areas and roadside edges, growing as a biennial plant.

4.3 Harvesting Techniques

- **Best Time to Harvest**: Late summer is optimal for collecting milk thistle seeds, where the concentration of silymarin is at its peak as the flower heads dry.

- **How to Harvest**: Wearing gloves to protect against the plant's spiny bracts is essential. Cut the flower heads, place them in a paper bag, and allow them to dry, shaking occasionally to loosen the seeds.

4.4 Preparation and Usage

- **Medicinal Preparations**: Milk thistle seeds can be ground and used in capsules or extracted into a tincture to maximize the bioavailability of silymarin, effectively delivering this powerful antioxidant.

- **Culinary Uses**: Though less common, the seeds can be roasted and ground as a coffee substitute, offering a mild, nutty flavor.

4.5 Contraindications and Cautions

- **Drug Interactions**: Milk thistle may interfere with the metabolism of certain drugs, such as allergy medications and blood thinners, due to its potent effect on liver enzymes.

- **Pregnancy and Breastfeeding**: Usage during these periods should be approached with caution; always consult a healthcare provider before beginning any new treatment.

4.6 Sustainable Foraging and Conservation

- **Environmental Impact**: Although sometimes considered invasive, responsible harvesting of milk thistle ensures that it does not disrupt local flora. Managing its spread in non-native areas is crucial to protect biodiversity.

Scientific Insights from Research:

A study highlighted in the *World Journal of Hepatology* provides a comprehensive look at silymarin's hepatoprotective effects. It explains that silymarin not only prevents liver damage by enhancing the antioxidant defense system but also by stimulating protein synthesis, which is crucial for liver repair. Moreover, silymarin's ability to block toxins from entering liver cells and its anti-inflammatory properties significantly contribute to its effectiveness in treating liver diseases (Vargas-Mendoza et al., 2014).

Chapter 5: Dandelion Root

Dandelion root, scientifically known as TARAXACUM OFFICINALE, is a perennial plant widely recognized for its extensive range of health benefits. From ancient remedies to modern applications, this chapter explores the rich medicinal properties of dandelion root, particularly focusing on its antioxidant, hepatoprotective, and anticancer activities. This discussion draws on a comprehensive review of its benefits published in the BULLETIN OF THE NATIONAL RESEARCH CENTRE by Di Napoli and Zucchetti (2021).

5.1 Medicinal Properties of Dandelion Root

- **Antioxidant Capacity**: Dandelion root is rich in several antioxidants, including flavonoids and phenolic acids like caffeic and chlorogenic acids. These compounds help to neutralize harmful free radicals in the body, reducing oxidative stress and preventing cellular damage. Studies have shown that these antioxidant properties extend to reducing inflammation and protecting against chronic diseases such as cardiovascular disease and diabetes.

- **Liver Health**: Dandelion root has been traditionally used to support liver function and detoxification. The review by Di Napoli and Zucchetti (2021) highlights its hepatoprotective properties, demonstrating that dandelion can effectively counteract liver damage caused by environmental toxins and dietary excesses. This protective effect is primarily due to its ability to enhance the natural antioxidant systems of the liver and support the regeneration of liver tissue.

- **Cancer Prevention and Treatment**: The same review points to emerging evidence that dandelion root may possess anticancer properties. This includes its potential to induce apoptosis (programmed cell death) in cancer cells without harming healthy cells. Notably, the root extract has shown effectiveness against several types of cancer, including leukemia and cancers of the breast, prostate, and colon.

5.2 Botanical Description and Habitat

- Dandelion is easily recognized by its bright yellow flowers and deeply toothed, lance-shaped leaves. It thrives across a wide range of habitats but prefers sunny and open environments. The plant is incredibly hardy, often found in urban lawns and

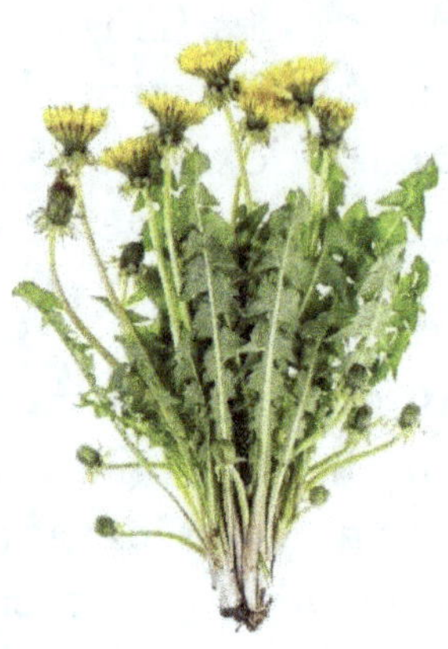

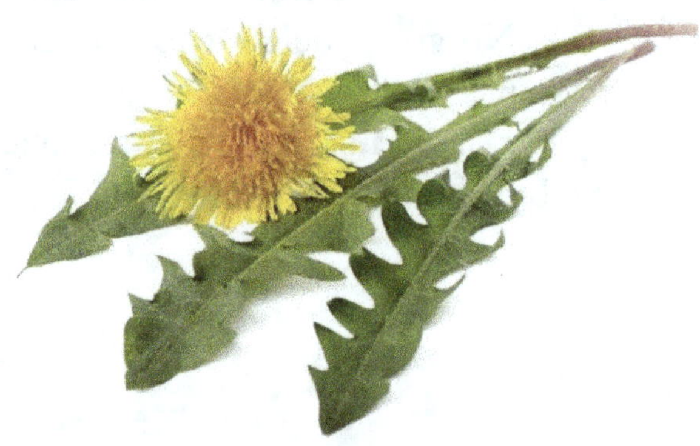

roadside verges as well as in meadows and pastures.

5.3 Harvesting and Usage

- The root of the dandelion is harvested in late fall when the plant's medicinal compounds are at their peak. It is typically dried and can be used to make teas, tinctures, or powders.

- Culinary uses of dandelion root include its use as a coffee substitute after roasting, or it can be added to soups and stews to impart a bitter yet enriching flavor.

5.4 Safety and Precautions

- While dandelion root is generally considered safe for most people, it can interact with certain medications, especially those affecting the liver. It is also a diuretic, which can affect the body's mineral balance.

- Individuals with allergies to ragweed and related plants may also react to dandelion.

5.5 Conservation and Sustainable Harvesting

- Given its status as a common weed in many parts of the world, dandelion does not generally face conservation pressures. However, sustainable harvesting practices should be maintained to ensure that local ecosystems are not disrupted.

5.6 Conclusion

The review by Di Napoli and Zucchetti (2021) provides compelling evidence of the broad therapeutic potential of TARAXACUM OFFICINALE, particularly highlighting its role in promoting liver health, combating oxidative stress, and offering anticancer benefits. Further research is encouraged to fully explore and validate these properties, ensuring dandelion's place in both traditional and modern medicinal practices.

REFERENCE: Di Napoli, A., & Zucchetti, P. (2021). A comprehensive review of the benefits of Taraxacum officinale on human health. BULLETIN OF THE NATIONAL RESEARCH CENTRE, 45(110). https://doi.org/10.1186/s42269-021-00567-1

Chapter 6: Plantain

Plantain, scientifically known as PLANTAGO MAJOR, is a perennial herb found across various climates and regions, widely acknowledged for its diverse medicinal properties. This chapter explores plantain's pharmacological effects, including its benefits for gastrointestinal and liver health, drawing on recent clinical studies and traditional uses.

6.1 Medicinal Properties of Plantain

- **Gastrointestinal Health**: Plantain seeds have shown promise in managing ulcerative colitis (UC), a chronic inflammatory bowel disease. A study by Karimi et al. (2021) demonstrated that patients consuming 3600 mg/day of roasted P. MAJOR seeds experienced significant improvements in symptoms such as abdominal tenderness, visible blood in stool, and gastroesophageal reflux, compared to those receiving a placebo. This suggests plantain's potential in complementing standard UC treatments.

- **Liver Health**: Another study highlighted plantain's role in improving liver enzymes in patients with nonalcoholic fatty liver disease (NAFLD). Participants receiving plantain supplementation showed notable reductions in liver enzymes like ALT and AST, which are indicative of liver health. This study underscores plantain's hepatoprotective properties and its potential to enhance liver function through its anti-inflammatory and antioxidant actions.

6.2 Botanical Description and Habitat

- Plantain features broad, oval leaves that are easily recognizable along pathways,

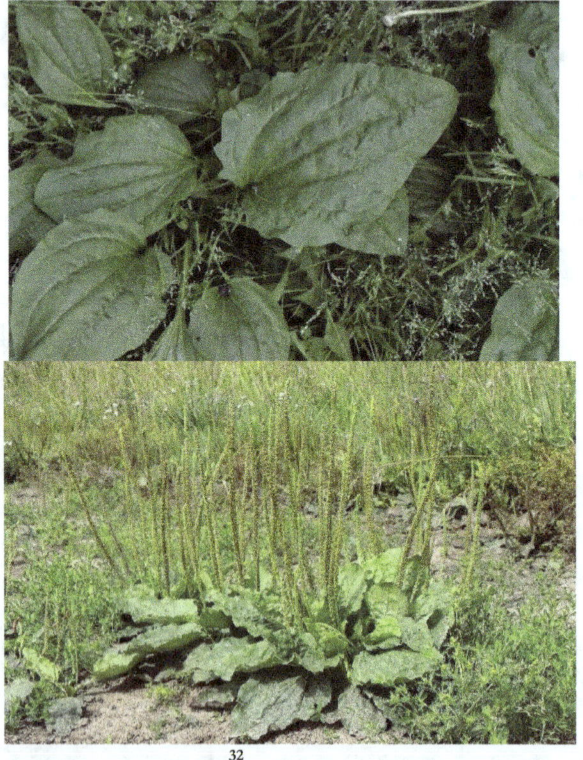

meadows, and garden edges. Its resilience and widespread distribution make it a common yet potent medicinal herb.

6.3 Harvesting and Usage

- **Best Time to Harvest**: The leaves and seeds of plantain can be harvested throughout its growing season, with late spring to early summer being ideal for leaves and late summer for seeds.

- **Culinary and Medicinal Preparations**: Plantain leaves can be used fresh in salads or dried for tea, which is soothing for digestive issues and skin irritations. The seeds are often used in powdered form or as a decoction.

6.4 Safety and Precautions

- **Interactions and Contraindications**: While plantain is generally safe, it can interact with medications due to its impact on digestive and liver enzymes. It's advised to consult healthcare providers before starting any new remedy, especially for individuals on medication for liver or digestive ailments.

6.5 Sustainable Foraging and Conservation

- Plantain's abundance makes it an ideal candidate for sustainable foraging. Collectors should ensure to leave enough plants for regeneration and to avoid overharvesting in any given area.

6.6 Scientific Insights and Future Research Directions

- The studies mentioned provide a scientific basis for plantain's traditional uses, particularly in gastrointestinal and liver health. Future research could explore its broader therapeutic potentials, including its full range of bioactive compounds. Further studies with larger sample sizes and long-term follow-up are needed to establish more detailed guidelines for its clinical use.

References:

- Karimi, G., et al. (2021). Efficacy of Plantago major seed in management of ulcerative colitis symptoms: A randomized, placebo-controlled, clinical trial. **Complementary Therapies in Clinical Practice, 44, 101444**.

- Jazayeri, S. F., et al. (2021). The Efficacy of Plantago major Seed on Liver Enzymes in Nonalcoholic Fatty Liver Disease: A Randomized Double-Blind Clinical Trial. **Evidence-Based Complementary and Alternative Medicine, 2021, Article ID 6693887**.

Chapter 7: Lactuca Virosa/Wild Lettuce

Wild lettuce, also known as opium lettuce because of its ability to relieve pain (without addiction, of course), known scientifically as *Lactuca virosa*, is a biennial plant widely recognized for its historical use as a mild sedative and pain reliever. This chapter explores the herb's medicinal properties, particularly focusing on its analgesic and sedative effects, and draws on recent scientific studies to underscore its potential benefits and applications.

7.1 Medicinal Properties of Wild Lettuce

- **Pain Relief and Sedative Effects**: Wild lettuce is best known for its sedative and analgesic properties, attributed to a milky substance called lactucarium, which the plant secretes. This substance contains compounds such as lactucin and lactucopicrin, which have been shown to possess analgesic and sedative activities. These effects make wild lettuce beneficial for treating various ailments, including insomnia, anxiety, and nervous restlessness. The study conducted by Abidet et al. (2020) noted that the ethyl acetate extract of

Lactuca virosa exhibited moderate antioxidant activity, which can contribute to its anti-inflammatory properties, supporting its use in pain management.

- **Antioxidant Activity**: The same study also highlighted the significant antioxidant potential of wild lettuce, with different extracts showing varying degrees of efficacy in scavenging free radicals. This activity is crucial as it helps reduce oxidative stress in the body, which is often associated with inflammation and pain.

7.2 Botanical Description and Habitat

- Wild lettuce typically grows to a height of up to six feet and features bright green

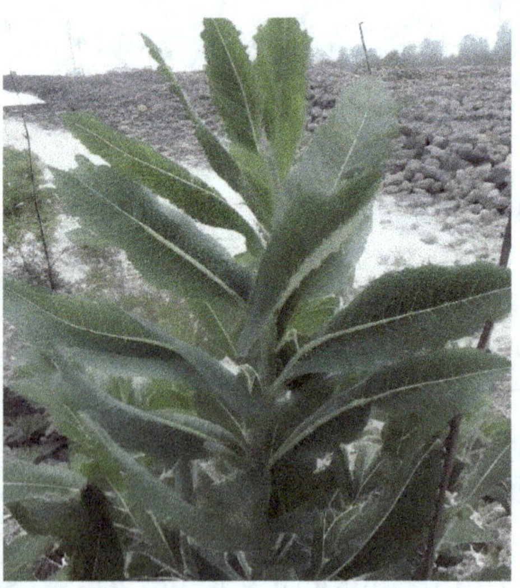

leaves and a sturdy, central stem that exudes a white, milky sap when cut. This plant prefers full sunlight and is commonly found along riverbanks and on the edges of fields and roads.

7.3 Harvesting and Usage

- **Best Time to Harvest**: The optimal time for harvesting wild lettuce for medicinal purposes is just before it flowers in early summer, when the content of lactucarium is highest.

- **Medicinal Preparations**: The leaves and stems can be dried and used to make a tea or tincture, which exploits the sedative properties of the plant. The dried sap can also be used directly in small amounts as a natural pain reliever.

7.4 Safety and Precautions

- **Usage Cautions**: While generally safe for most people in moderate amounts, wild lettuce should be used with caution due to its potent sedative effects, which can vary greatly depending on the dosage and the individual's response.

- **Potential Side Effects**: Excessive use can lead to symptoms such as dizziness, nausea, and, in extreme cases, difficulty breathing due to its thoracic suppression capabilities.

7.5 Sustainable Foraging and Conservation

- As wild lettuce can grow abundantly in suitable conditions, sustainable harvesting involves taking only what is necessary and ensuring that plants are not uprooted completely, allowing them to regenerate and spread naturally.

7.6 Conclusion

The recent studies, including the findings from Abidet et al. (2020), provide valuable insights into the pharmacological potential of wild lettuce, especially its role in pain management and as a natural sedative. These findings support the traditional uses of wild lettuce and open avenues for its potential therapeutic applications, highlighting the need for further research to fully understand its efficacy and safety profile.

References:

- Abidet, A., Gherraf, N., Kalla, A., Zellagui, A., & Fella, O. (2020). Assessment of total phenolics and flavonoids, and evaluation of scavenging activity of the aerial parts of *Verbascum thapsus L.* and *Lactuca virosa L.* grown in Algeria. *International Journal of Chemical and Biochemical Sciences*, 17, 86-92.

7.7 A Special Note

Distinguishing Between Plantain and Wild Lettuce

While plantain (PLANTAGO MAJOR) and wild lettuce (LACTUCA VIROSA) may share similar environments and have overlapping traditional uses, they are distinctly different in appearance, habitat preferences, and certain medicinal properties. Here's a detailed comparison to help foragers and herbal enthusiasts correctly identify and utilize each plant:

Plantain (Plantago major)

- **Appearance**: Plantain has broad, oval leaves that grow in a rosette at the base of the plant. The leaves are smooth and feature prominent parallel veins. It produces a flower spike that is not branched, with tiny white flowers that encircle the spike.

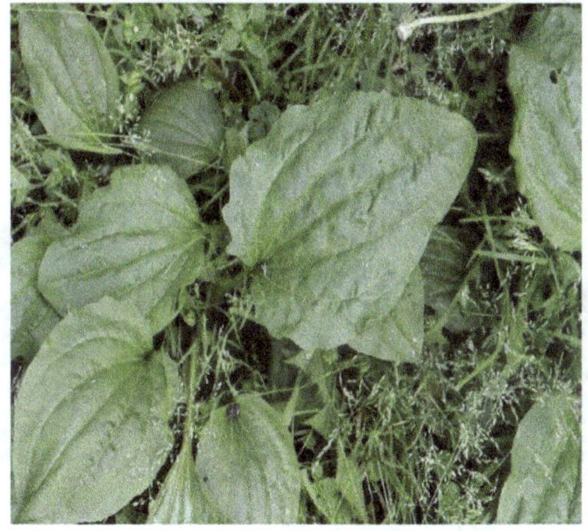

- **Habitat**: Thrives in compacted soils and is commonly found in paths, lawns, and other areas subject to frequent disturbance. Plantain prefers a slightly more shaded environment compared to wild lettuce.

- **Medicinal Uses**: Known for its wound-healing abilities due to the presence of allantoin. It is also used for its anti-inflammatory, antimicrobial, and mild analgesic properties. Plantain can be particularly effective in soothing digestive issues and is used in treating respiratory problems.

Wild Lettuce (Lactuca virosa)

- **Appearance**: Wild lettuce is taller and more upright, with a central stem that can grow up to six feet tall. The leaves are

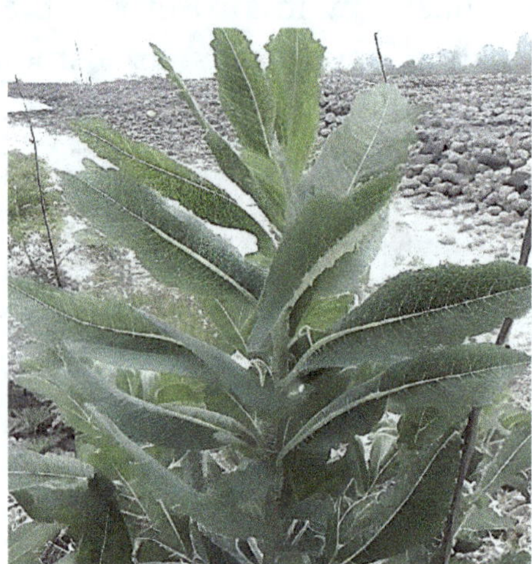

elongated, lobed, and have a slightly prickly texture. A key identifying feature is the milky sap (lactucarium) that exudes from the stem when it is broken.

- **Habitat**: Prefers full sun and is often found along riverbanks, along roadsides, and in fields. Wild lettuce can grow in less compacted soil than plantain and typically seeks more open, sunnier spaces.

- **Medicinal Uses**: The lactucarium in wild lettuce is known for its sedative and pain-relieving properties, making it beneficial for treating insomnia, anxiety, and pain. It is also used for its antitussive (cough suppressant) effects.

Foraging Tips to Differentiate:

1. **Leaf Structure**: Plantain's broad, flat leaves with parallel veins are quite distinct from the more ragged, serrated leaves of wild lettuce that contain a central vein with branching smaller veins.

2. **Sap Color**: Breaking the stem of wild lettuce will reveal a white, milky sap, whereas plantain does not produce any milky sap.

3. **Flower Shape and Arrangement**: Plantain's flowers are small, inconspicuous, and tightly packed along a spike, whereas wild lettuce has small yellow or pale blue flower heads that form a loose cluster.

Understanding these differences is crucial for proper identification and use, especially when foraging for medicinal purposes. By recognizing each plant's unique characteristics, foragers can ensure they are using the right plant for the right remedy.

Chapter 8: Nettles

Nettles, scientifically referred to as URTICA DIOICA, are perennial flowering plants with a wealth of medicinal properties and nutritional value. This chapter delves into the diverse varieties of nettles and their specific health benefits, supported by the latest scientific research.

8.1 Medicinal Properties of Nettles

- **Nutritional and Antioxidant Properties**: Nettles are highly nutritious, containing significant levels of vitamins A, C, and E, and minerals such as iron, magnesium, and calcium. The antioxidant properties of nettles contribute to reducing oxidative stress and inflammation, which is beneficial in preventing chronic diseases like diabetes and hypertension.

- **Anti-diabetic Properties**: Studies have shown that nettles possess antidiabetic properties due to their ability to modulate blood glucose levels. They enhance insulin secretion and the regeneration of pancreatic beta cells, crucial for managing diabetes. This action is partly due to the flavonoids they contain, such as quercetin, which has been found to improve the lipid profile and decrease blood sugar levels.

- **Antihypertensive Effects**: Nettles are known for their ability to lower blood pressure, an essential factor in cardiovascular health. This effect is mediated through various mechanisms, including direct vasodilatory effects facilitated by nitric oxide release and the inhibition of calcium channels, which helps in relaxing blood vessels.

8.2 Botanical Description and Varieties

- Nettles are typically characterized by their 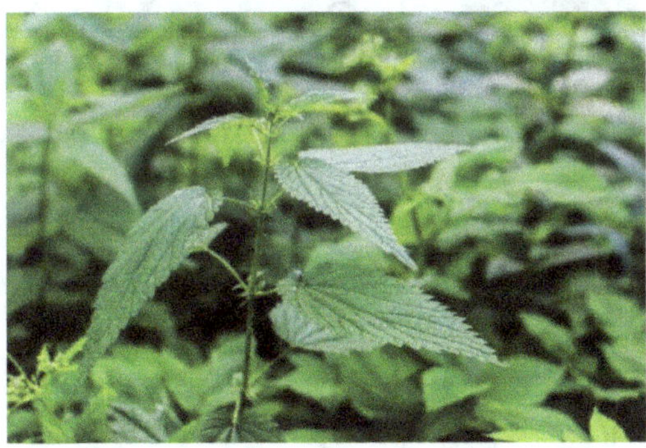 heart-shaped, serrated leaves covered with tiny hairs that can sting, giving them the common name "stinging nettles." They flourish in nitrogen-rich soil and are commonly found in Europe, North America, parts of Africa, and Asia.

- **Varieties**: There are several species of nettles, each with unique characteristics and uses. For example, URTICA DIOICA is the most widely known, but other species like LAPORTEA ALATIPES and OBETIA TENAX are studied for their specific health benefits, particularly in traditional African medicine.

8.3 Harvesting and Usage

• **Optimal Harvesting Time**: The best time to harvest nettles is in spring when the leaves are young and tender, making them ideal for consumption and rich in nutrients.

- **Preparations**: Nettles can be used in various forms—dried for teas, cooked like spinach, or as extracts for supplements. Cooking nettles removes their sting, making them safe to eat.

8.4 Safety and Precautions

- **Interactions**: Despite their health benefits, nettles can interact with certain medications like blood thinners, blood pressure medications, and diuretics due to their potent effects on blood and metabolism.

- **Allergic Reactions**: Individuals sensitive to nettle or similar plants should use them cautiously to avoid allergic reactions.

8.5 Conservation and Sustainable Foraging

- Given their ability to grow aggressively, sustainable harvesting practices are essential to ensure that nettles are collected in ways that do not harm the environment. Foragers should harvest nettles in moderation and from areas where they are abundant.

8.6 Conclusion

Recent studies, including those from the Pharmaceutical Research Center at Mashhad University, have highlighted nettles' potential in treating complex syndromes like metabolic syndrome by addressing multiple symptoms simultaneously, such as high blood pressure, high sugar levels, and lipid imbalances. This robust body of research supports the traditional uses of nettles and underscores their potential in modern herbal medicine and nutrition.

References:

- Mahlangeni, N. T., et al. (2020). Nutritional value, antioxidant and antidiabetic properties of nettles. SCIENTIFIC REPORTS, 10, 9762. https://doi.org/10.1038/s41598-020-67055-w

- Samakar, B., et al. (2022). A review of the effects of URTICA DIOICA (nettle) in metabolic syndrome. IRANIAN JOURNAL OF BASIC MEDICAL SCIENCES, 25, 543-553. https://dx.doi.org/10.22038/IJBMS.2022.58892.13079

•

Chapter 9: Chamomile

Chamomile, known for its soothing and healing properties, is one of the most ancient medicinal herbs. This chapter explores the extensive uses and benefits of two primary species of chamomile: German chamomile (MATRICARIA CHAMOMILLA) and Roman chamomile (CHAMAEMELUM NOBILE), supported by scientific research.

9.1 Medicinal Properties of Chamomile

- **Anti-inflammatory and Antioxidant Properties**: Chamomile is renowned for its potent anti-inflammatory and antioxidant capabilities. These properties are attributed to its rich content of flavonoids like apigenin, which has been shown to reduce inflammation and combat oxidative stress, thereby preventing cell damage.

- **Sedative and Anti-anxiety Effects**: Both German and Roman chamomile are used for their sedative effects, helping to alleviate anxiety, promote relaxation, and improve sleep quality. These effects are particularly attributed to the flavonoid apigenin, which binds to benzodiazepine receptors in the brain, mimicking the effects of tranquilizers.

- **Gastrointestinal Relief**: Chamomile is effective in soothing gastrointestinal disturbances, including indigestion, motion sickness, nausea, and vomiting, due to its antispasmodic and carminative properties.

9.2 Botanical Description and Habitat

- **German Chamomile**: This annual herb features daisy-like white flowers with yellow centers and feathery leaves. It primarily grows in Europe and

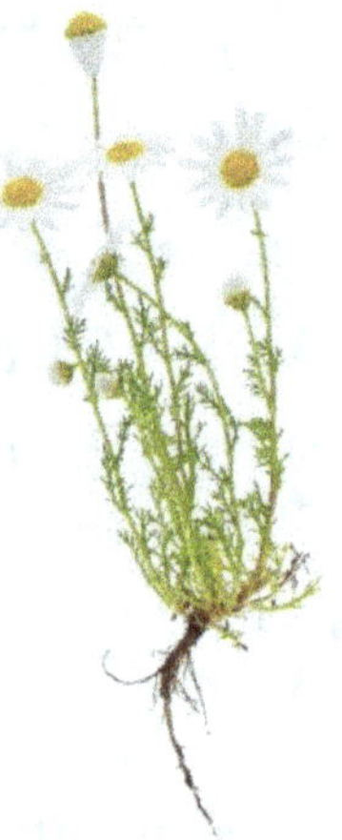

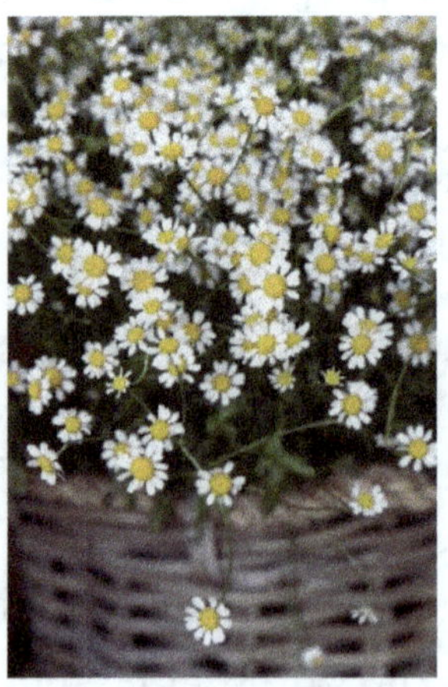

parts of Asia but has been widely naturalized around the world.

- **Roman Chamomile**: A perennial plant, Roman chamomile has similar daisy-like flowers but grows closer to the ground, often used as a

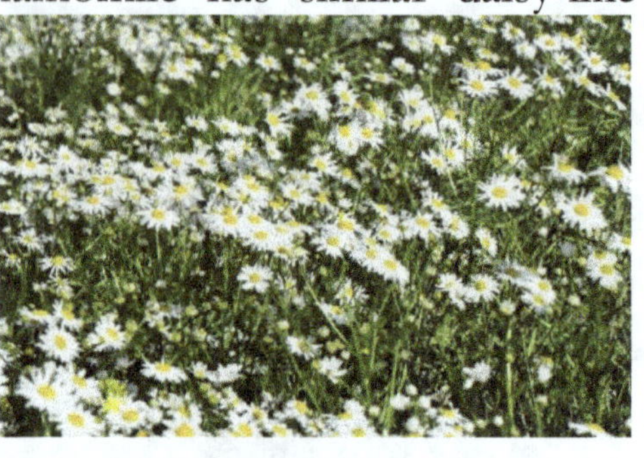

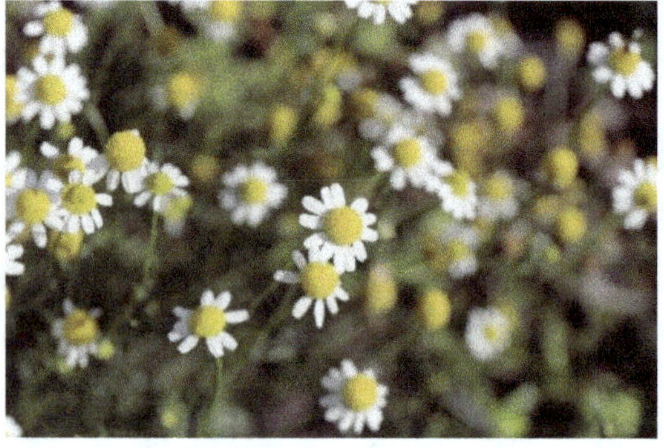

ground cover. It emits a more intense and sweeter aroma compared to its German counterpart.

9.3 Harvesting and Usage

- **Harvesting**: The flowers of both species are harvested in summer when they are in full bloom, as the active ingredients are most potent during this time.

- **Usage**: Chamomile is commonly used in teas, tinctures, and topical applications. The dried flowers are steeped to make a soothing tea, which is widely consumed for its health benefits.

9.4 Safety and Precautions

- While generally safe, chamomile can cause allergic reactions in individuals sensitive to plants in the daisy family. It should be used cautiously by those on anticoagulant medications due to its potential to enhance their effects.

9.5 Conservation and Sustainable Harvesting

- Chamomile is abundant in the wild but should be harvested sustainably to ensure it does not deplete local stocks. Harvesters are encouraged to leave enough plants to allow for natural regeneration.

9.6 Conclusion

Recent research has supported the traditional uses of chamomile, confirming its role as a therapeutic agent for a variety of conditions due to its anti-inflammatory, antioxidant, and sedative properties . Future studies are expected to delve deeper into its potential, broadening the scope of its applications in both traditional and modern medicine.

References:

- Sah, A. et al. (2022). A Comprehensive Study of Therapeutic Applications of Chamomile. PHARMACEUTICALS, 15(1284). https://doi.org/10.3390/ph15101284

Chapter 10: Elderberry

Elderberry, renowned for its medicinal properties, has been utilized in traditional remedies for centuries. This chapter explores the benefits of elderberry, particularly focusing on its use in treating and preventing viral respiratory infections and its potent antioxidant activities, supported by scientific research.

10.1 Medicinal Properties of Elderberry

- **Antiviral Properties**: Elderberry is known for its antiviral capabilities against various strains of influenza and potentially other viral respiratory pathogens. Compounds within elderberry, such as flavonoids, appear to inhibit the early stages of infection by blocking key viral proteins responsible for attachment and entry into host cells.

- **Immune System Modulation**: Elderberry has an immunomodulating effect, increasing the production of cytokines which are crucial for the immune system's response to infection. While concerns have been raised about the potential for a 'cytokine storm,' particularly related to COVID-19, current evidence suggests that elderberry does not exacerbate this condition and may actually play a beneficial role in managing inflammation.

- **Reduction in Cold and Flu Symptoms**: Studies suggest that elderberry can reduce the duration and severity of influenza and common cold symptoms. This effect is attributed to its antiviral properties and immune-enhancing effects, which help the body combat and recover from illness more quickly.

10.2 Botanical Description and Habitat

- **Species Varieties**: Elderberry includes multiple species, most notably SAMBUCUS NIGRA (European elderberry) and SAMBUCUS CANADENSIS (American elderberry). Both species are used similarly in medicinal preparations, although the European variety is more extensively studied and utilized in commercial products.

- **Physical Characteristics**: Elderberry plants are characterized by their clusters of small, white to cream flowers and dark purple to black berries.

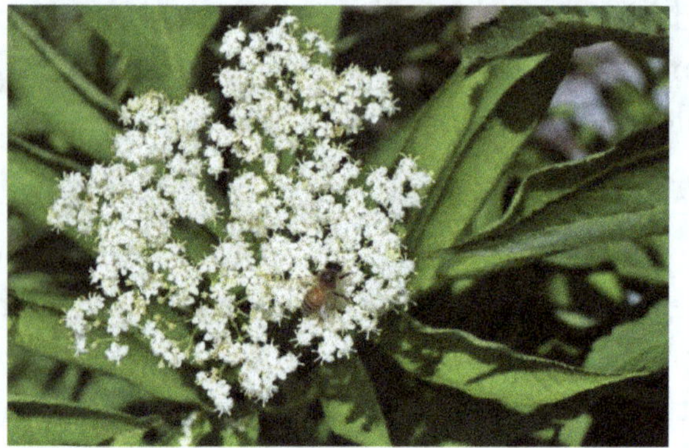

They are deciduous shrubs or small trees that grow well in a variety of conditions but prefer moist, well-drained soils.

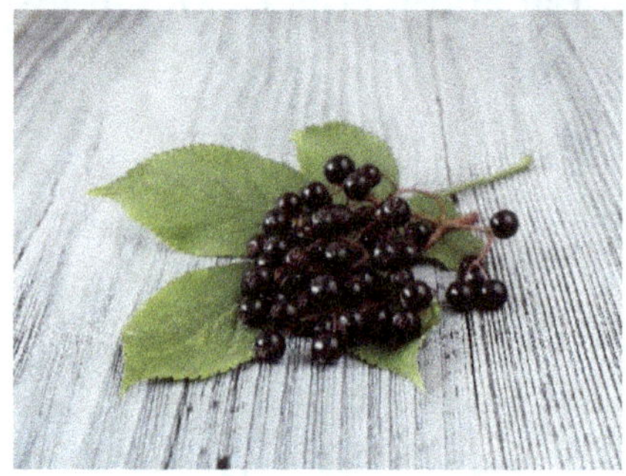

10.3 Harvesting and Usage

- **Harvesting**: The flowers and berries of the elderberry plant are the parts most commonly used for medicinal purposes. Berries should be picked when fully ripe and typically processed immediately to preserve their medicinal qualities.

- **Usage:** Elderberry is available in various forms, including syrups, gummies, lozenges, and teas. It is widely used both for immune system enhancement and as a treatment for acute viral infections.

10.4 Safety and Precautions

- Elderberry is generally safe when used appropriately. However, uncooked or raw berries, leaves, bark, and roots of the plant contain compounds that can be toxic, so commercial preparations or proper home processing is crucial.

10.5 Conservation and Sustainable Harvesting

- While elderberry plants are abundant and robust, sustainable harvesting practices are recommended to ensure that wild populations are not depleted. Cultivation of elderberry for commercial use is increasing, reflecting its growing popularity as a health supplement.

10.6 Conclusion

Elderberry's role in traditional and modern medicine continues to be supported by emerging scientific research, particularly in the areas of immune modulation and antiviral effects. While further research is needed to fully understand its benefits and limitations, elderberry remains a valuable component of natural health and wellness strategies.

References:

- Wieland, L.S., et al. (2021). Elderberry for prevention and treatment of viral respiratory illnesses: a systematic review. BMC COMPLEMENTARY MEDICINE AND THERAPIES, 21(112). https://doi.org/10.1186/s12906-021-03283-5

- Charlebois, D. (2007). Elderberry as a medicinal plant. In ISSUES IN NEW CROPS AND NEW USES (pp. 284-292). ASHS Press, Alexandria, VA.

Chapter 11: Yarrow

Yarrow, known botanically as ACHILLEA MILLEFOLIUM, is a perennial herb renowned for its extensive medicinal properties. This chapter dives into the specific benefits of yarrow, including its anti-inflammatory, antibacterial, and wound-healing effects, bolstered by scientific findings.

11.1 Medicinal Properties of Yarrow

- **Anti-inflammatory and Wound Healing**: Yarrow is traditionally used for its anti-inflammatory properties and ability to promote wound healing. It contains flavonoids and sesquiterpene lactones, which contribute to its ability to reduce inflammation and aid in skin regeneration. Studies have demonstrated its effectiveness in treating inflammatory skin conditions and speeding up the healing process of wounds.

- **Antibacterial Effects**: Yarrow exhibits significant antibacterial activities, particularly against HELICOBACTER PYLORI, a bacterium associated with several gastrointestinal diseases. This effect is attributed to its rich profile of phenolic compounds, which disrupt bacterial cell membranes and inhibit bacterial growth.

- **Gastrointestinal Health**: Yarrow has been shown to improve gastrointestinal health by reducing gastrointestinal inflammation and potentially treating ulcers. Its application in traditional medicine includes treatment for irritable bowel syndrome and other inflammatory bowel diseases.

11.2 Botanical Description and Habitat

- Yarrow is characterized by its feathery foliage and clusters of small, white to pink flowers. It

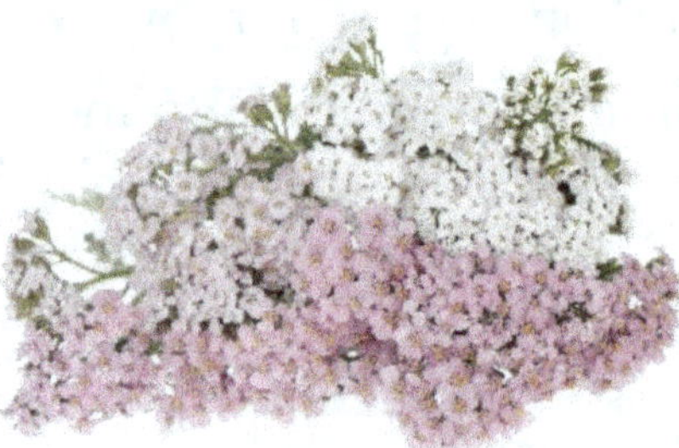

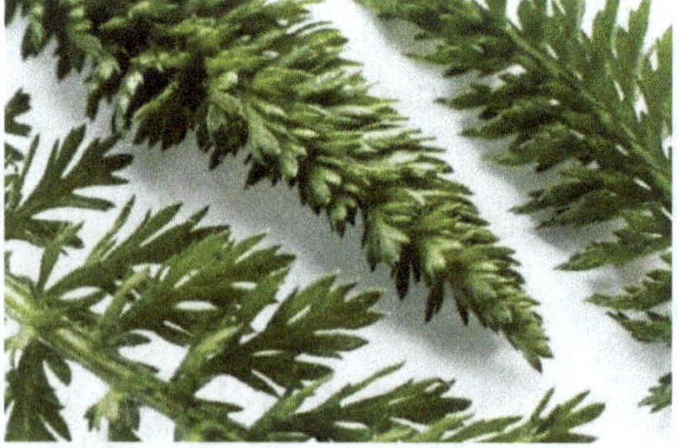

is commonly found in the temperate regions of the Northern Hemisphere in meadows, roadsides, and open forests.

11.3 Harvesting and Usage

- **Harvesting**: The best time to harvest yarrow is during its flowering season in the summer when its medicinal compounds are most potent.

- **Usage**: Yarrow can be used in various forms, including teas, tinctures, and topical ointments. It is often applied directly to the skin for wounds and used internally for its anti-inflammatory and antibacterial benefits.

11.4 Safety and Precautions

- Yarrow is generally safe but can cause allergic reactions in people sensitive to the Asteraceae family. It should be used with caution by those on anticoagulant therapy as it can potentially increase the risk of bleeding.

11.5 Conservation and Sustainable Harvesting

- While yarrow is abundant, it is crucial to harvest it sustainably to avoid depleting local populations and maintain its availability in natural habitats.

11.6 Conclusion

Research supports the traditional uses of yarrow for its anti-inflammatory, antibacterial, and wound-healing properties, making it a valuable herb in natural medicine for treating a wide range of conditions.

References:

- Villalva, M., et al. (2022). Antioxidant, Anti-Inflammatory, and Antibacterial Properties of an Achillea millefolium L. Extract. ANTIOXIDANTS, 11, 1849. https://doi.org/10.3390/antiox11101849

- Yakhkeshi, S., et al. (2012). Effects of Yarrow on Immune Response and Serum Lipids in Broilers. JOURNAL OF AGRICULTURAL SCIENCE AND TECHNOLOGY, 14, 799-810. https://sid.ir/2471

Chapter 12: Burdock

Burdock is celebrated for its nutritional value and medicinal properties, especially known for its role in detoxification and digestive health. This chapter delves into the scientifically supported benefits of burdock root, including its efficacy in treating gastrointestinal disorders and enhancing overall health.

12.1 Medicinal Properties of Burdock

- **Gastrointestinal Health**: Burdock root is highly valued for its ability to repair gastrointestinal mucosa and manage peptic ulcers, largely due to its anti-inflammatory and antibacterial properties. Studies have shown that burdock can significantly reduce the size of gastric ulcers and effectively eradicate Helicobacter pylori infections, a common cause of gastric issues.

- **Antioxidant and Anti-inflammatory Properties**: Burdock root is rich in antioxidants such as quercetin and luteolin, which help mitigate oxidative stress and reduce inflammation throughout the body.

These compounds are particularly effective in supporting liver health and promoting blood purification.

- **Diuretic and Detoxifying Effects**: The root promotes urine production and helps in the elimination of waste from the body. This diuretic effect supports kidney function and detoxifies the liver, enhancing overall health and wellness.

12.2 Botanical Description and Habitat

- Burdock is a biennial plant characterized by

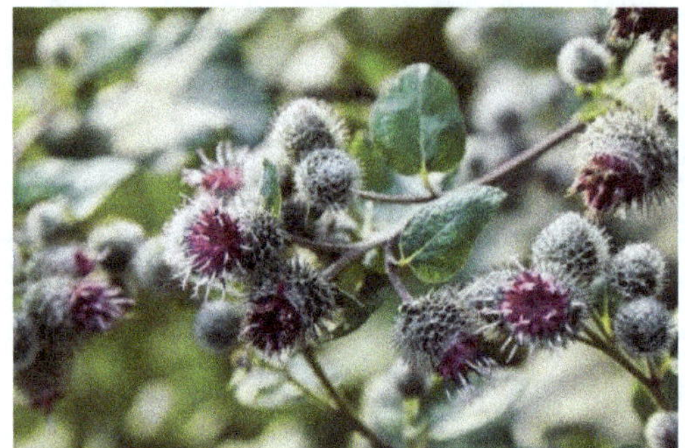

its broad leaves and prickly heads. The plant thrives in a variety of soil types, though it prefers well-drained soil.

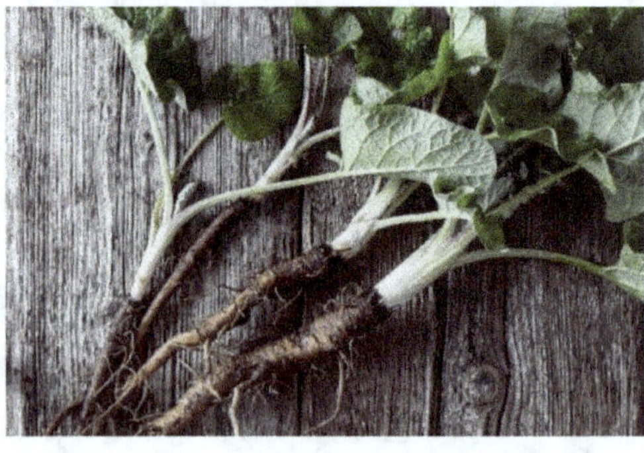

12.3 Harvesting and Usage

- **Harvesting**: The roots are best harvested in their first year of growth when they are young and tender. Mature roots can become woody and less palatable.

- **Usage**: Burdock root can be eaten raw, cooked, or dried and used in teas. It is also processed into supplements such as capsules and tinctures for medicinal use.

12.4 Safety and Precautions

- While generally safe for most people, burdock should be used cautiously by those with allergies to other members of the daisy family. It's also advised to consult with a healthcare provider before using burdock as it can interact with medications, particularly those for diabetes and blood clotting.

12.5 Conservation and Sustainable Harvesting

- Despite its robust nature, sustainable harvesting practices are recommended to ensure that wild populations are not threatened. Cultivating burdock in a controlled environment can help meet demand without overharvesting wild stocks.

12.6 Conclusion

Research underscores the therapeutic potential of burdock, particularly in treating gastrointestinal ailments and enhancing detoxification pathways. With its nutritional and medicinal benefits, burdock remains a valuable herb in natural medicine practices.

References:

- Wu et al. (2010). Burdock Essence Promotes Gastrointestinal Mucosal Repair in Ulcer Patients. FOOYIN JOURNAL OF HEALTH SCIENCES, 2(1), 26-31.

- Moro, T.M.A., & Clerici, M.T.P.S. (2021). Burdock (Arctium lappa L.) roots as a source of inulin-type fructans and other bioactive compounds. FOOD RESEARCH INTERNATIONAL, 141, 109889. https://doi.org/10.1016/j.foodres.2020.109889

Chapter 13: Lemon Balm (Melissa)

Lemon balm, or *Melissa officinalis*, is a perennial herb that is treasured for its wide range of health benefits. This chapter will delve into the detailed medicinal properties, botanical characteristics, usage, safety, and conservation of lemon balm, integrating the latest research findings.

13.1 Medicinal Properties of Lemon Balm

- **Cognitive and Mood Enhancement**: Lemon balm is recognized for its cognitive and mood-enhancing effects. Studies have demonstrated its ability to improve memory and reduce stress, potentially offering benefits in the management of Alzheimer's disease due to its cholinergic activity.

- **Antioxidant and Anti-inflammatory Properties**: The plant's high phenolic content, including rosmarinic acid and flavonoids such as quercitrin and luteolin, contribute to its strong antioxidant and anti-inflammatory activities. These properties help in preventing oxidative stress-related diseases like cardiovascular diseases and cancers.

- **Antimicrobial and Antiviral Effects**: Lemon balm has shown antimicrobial and antiviral effects, including activity against herpes simplex virus and potentially HIV-1. This makes it useful in treating and managing conditions associated with these pathogens.

13.2 Botanical Description and Habitat

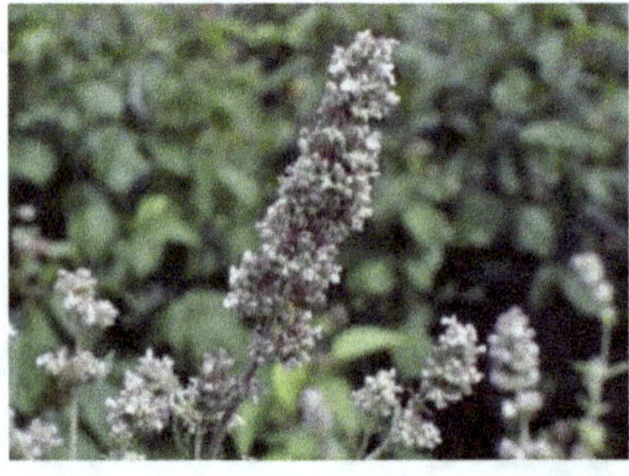

- Lemon balm typically grows in sandy and scrubby areas but is also found in damp wasteland at varying elevations. It features small, light pink or white flowers and broad, ovate leaves

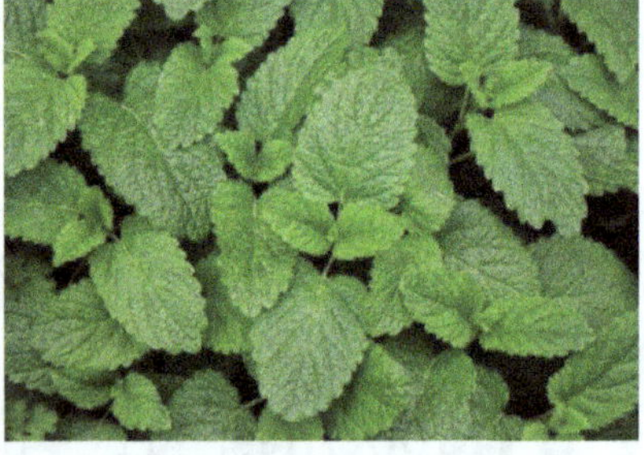

that emit a mild lemon scent when crushed.

13.3 Harvesting and Usage

- **Harvesting**: The leaves are best harvested just before or during the flowering stage when the essential oils and medicinal compounds are most potent.

- **Usage**: In lemon balm (*Melissa officinalis*), the leaves are the primary edible parts of the plant. They are commonly used both for culinary and medicinal purposes. The leaves have a mild lemon scent, which makes them a delightful addition to a variety of dishes and drinks.

Here are a few ways in which lemon balm leaves can be utilized:

1. **Culinary Uses**:

    o **Teas**: Lemon balm leaves are often steeped in hot water to make a soothing herbal tea.

    o **Salads**: Fresh leaves can be chopped and added to salads for a citrusy flavor.

    o **Soups and Sauces**: The leaves can be used as a seasoning in soups and sauces.

    o **Desserts**: Lemon balm can be infused into desserts for flavoring, such as ice creams, custards, and cakes.

2. **Medicinal Uses**:

- o **Tinctures and Extracts**: The leaves are used to make tinctures and extracts which are believed to have calming and digestive benefits.

- o **Aromatherapy**: The essential oils from lemon balm leaves are used in aromatherapy for stress relief and relaxation.

The flowers of lemon balm, which are small and white, are also edible and can be used similarly to the leaves, though they are less commonly utilized. The primary focus for both culinary and medicinal uses remains the leaves due to their rich flavor and beneficial properties.

13.4 Safety and Precautions

- Generally considered safe for most people, lemon balm should be used cautiously by those on thyroid medication or sedatives due to potential interactions. It is also advised to avoid use during pregnancy and lactation without medical advice.

13.5 Conservation and Sustainable Harvesting

- Although lemon balm is abundant, sustainable harvesting practices are important to maintain wild populations and ensure ecological balance.

13.6 Conclusion

Lemon balm offers a variety of therapeutic benefits that make it a valuable plant in both traditional and modern medicine. Its potential in enhancing cognitive function and mood, alongside its antioxidant and antimicrobial properties, underscores its relevance in contemporary health treatments.

References:

- Kennedy, D. O. et al. (2003). Modulation of Mood and Cognitive Performance Following Acute Administration of Melissa Officinalis. *Neuropsychopharmacology*, 28, 1871–1881.

- Virchea, L.-I. et al. (2021). Phytochemical Analysis and Antioxidant Assay of Melissa Officinalis L. *Bio Web of Conferences*, 40.

- Ullah, M. A. et al. (2022). Medicinal Benefits of Lemon Balm (Melissa officinalis) for Human Health. *World Journal of Chemical and Pharmaceutical Sciences*, 01(01), 028–033.

Chapter 14: Peppermint

Peppermint, known scientifically as *Mentha piperita*, is a perennial herb acclaimed for its vibrant scent and cooling properties. This chapter explores the extensive medicinal benefits of peppermint, highlighting its therapeutic uses backed by scientific studies.

14.1 Medicinal Properties of Peppermint

- **Digestive Health**: Peppermint is highly effective in soothing gastrointestinal issues, notably irritable bowel syndrome (IBS). Its antispasmodic properties help relax the muscles of the intestines, easing the symptoms of IBS and reducing abdominal pain .

- **Respiratory Relief**: The menthol in peppermint acts as a decongestant, helping to clear the respiratory tract and provide relief from coughs, colds, and bronchial asthma.

- **Antimicrobial and Antiviral Effects**: Peppermint oil demonstrates significant antimicrobial and antiviral activities, making it effective against a variety of pathogens, including the herpes simplex virus and potentially inhibitory against the novel coronavirus (COVID-19) by disrupting virus-host interactions .

- **Neurological Benefits**: The aroma of peppermint has been found to enhance memory and increase alertness, providing a non-invasive way to boost cognitive function.

- **Pain Relief**: Peppermint is a natural analgesic and provides relief from headaches, muscular pains, and menstrual cramps due to its cooling menthol effect.

14.2 Botanical Description and Habitat

- Peppermint is characterized by its square stem, fast-growing leaves, and purple blooming

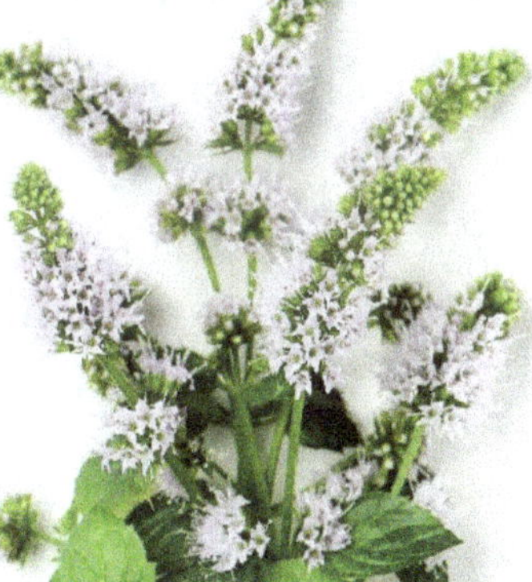

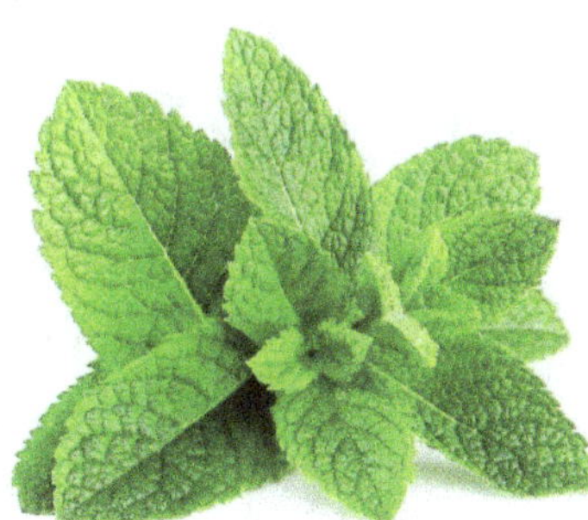

flowers. It thrives in moist, shaded locations but is adaptable to various environments.

14.3 Harvesting and Usage

- **Harvesting**: The leaves and oil of peppermint are harvested when the oil content is highest, just before flowering.

- **Usage**: Peppermint can be used fresh or dried in teas, culinary dishes, or extracted into oil for medicinal purposes.

14.4 Safety and Precautions

- While generally safe, peppermint should be used cautiously in people with gastroesophageal reflux disease (GERD) or those on medications metabolized by the liver, as it can exacerbate symptoms and affect drug metabolism.

14.5 Conservation and Sustainable Harvesting

- Peppermint is widely cultivated and does not generally face conservation issues; however, sustainable farming practices are encouraged to maintain soil health and biodiversity.

14.6 Conclusion

This chapter underlines the potency of peppermint as a medicinal plant with diverse applications in healthcare. Its benefits range from digestive health support to respiratory relief and pain alleviation, making it a valuable component in both herbal medicine and conventional treatment strategies.

References:

- Shabbir et al. (2020). Peppermint Oil, Its Useful, and Adverse Effects on Human Health: A Review. Innovare Journal of Ayurvedic Science.

- Chakraborty et al. (2022). Bioactive components of peppermint (Mentha piperita L.), their pharmacological and ameliorative potential and ethnomedicinal benefits: A review. Journal of Pharmacognosy and Phytochemistry.

Chapter 15: Crafting Topical Herbal Applications

This chapter guides you through the process of making topical applications using herbs renowned for their skin-healing properties. Here, we'll explore different methods and recipes for creating salves, balms, and poultices that harness the potent benefits of herbs like plantain, calendula, and chamomile.

Crafting Herbal Salves and Balms

- **Ingredients:**
    - 1 part dried herbal mixture (e.g., plantain, calendula, chamomile)
    - 5 parts carrier oil (e.g., coconut oil, almond oil, or olive oil)
    - 1 part beeswax (for salves) or shea butter (for balms)
- **Method:**

1. **Infuse the Oil**: Place the dried herbs and carrier oil in a double boiler. Gently heat for 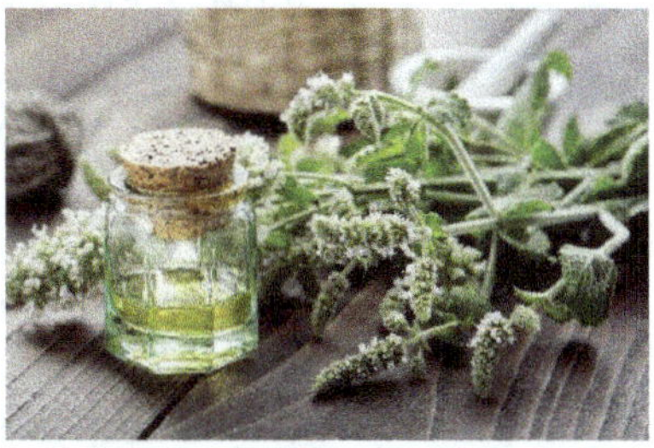 2-3 hours to allow the herbs to infuse into the oil, making sure not to burn the oil.

2. **Strain the Oil**: After infusion, strain the oil using cheesecloth to remove all plant matter. Ensure the oil is clear to prevent spoilage.

3. **Add Beeswax/Shea Butter**: Return the strained oil to the double boiler and add beeswax or shea butter. Heat until the beeswax or butter is completely melted, stirring to combine.

4. **Cool and Set**: Pour the mixture into clean containers and allow to cool and set. Once solidified, the salve or balm is ready to use.

Creating Herbal Poultices

- **Ingredients:**

- o Fresh or rehydrated herbs (e.g., plantain leaves, chamomile flowers)

- o Warm water (if using dried herbs)

- **Method:**

    1. **Prepare the Herbs**: If using dried herbs, rehydrate them with a little warm water until they are pliable. If using fresh herbs, crush them lightly to release their juices.

    2. **Apply**: Place the prepared herbs directly on the skin over the affected area. If the herb is very moist, it can be placed between two layers of cloth before applying to protect clothing or bedding.

    3. **Secure**: Use a bandage or a wrap to hold the poultice in place. Leave it on for 1-2 hours or as recommended.

    4. **Clean Up**: After removing the poultice, wash the area with warm water and pat dry.

Topical Infusions for Baths

- **Ingredients:**

    - o A handful of dried herbs (e.g., lavender, chamomile)

- o Large pot of boiling water

- **Method:**

  1. **Steep the Herbs**: Add the dried herbs to a pot of boiling water and remove from heat. Cover and let steep for 15-20 minutes.

  2. **Strain and Add to Bath**: Strain the infusion and add the herbal water to a warm bath.

  3. **Enjoy the Bath**: Soak in the bath for 20-30 minutes to allow the herbal properties to soothe the skin and relax the body.

These herbal preparations offer a natural way to soothe, heal, and nourish the skin using the powerful properties of herbs. Whether you're dealing with skin irritations, wounds, or just need a relaxing bath, these herbal topicals can provide effective and enjoyable benefits.

Chapter 16: Preparing Herbal Teas

Herbal teas, or tisanes, offer a delightful and therapeutic way to enjoy the benefits of herbs. This chapter explores 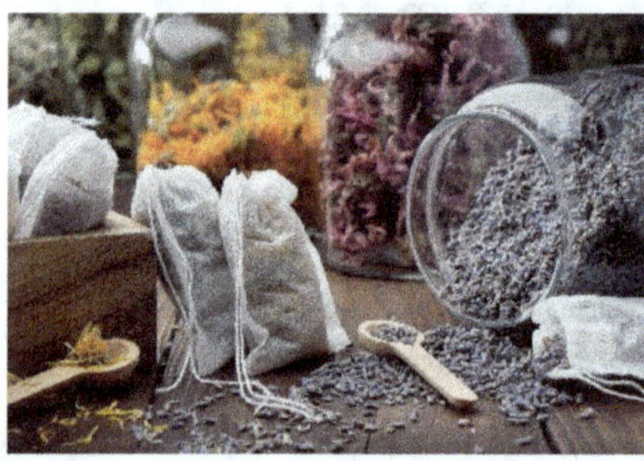 how to prepare herbal teas using the herbs discussed in this guide, with an emphasis on techniques that extract their maximum flavor and medicinal properties.

16.1 Preparing Herbal Teas

- **Ingredients**: Fresh or dried herbs (e.g., chamomile, peppermint, lemon balm)

- **Tools**: Teapot or infuser, kettle for boiling water

16.2 Basic Tea Making Steps

1. **Boil Water**: Start with fresh, cold water and bring it to a boil. The temperature of the water may need to be adjusted depending on the herb used (e.g., boiling for black tea, slightly cooler for delicate herbs like chamomile).

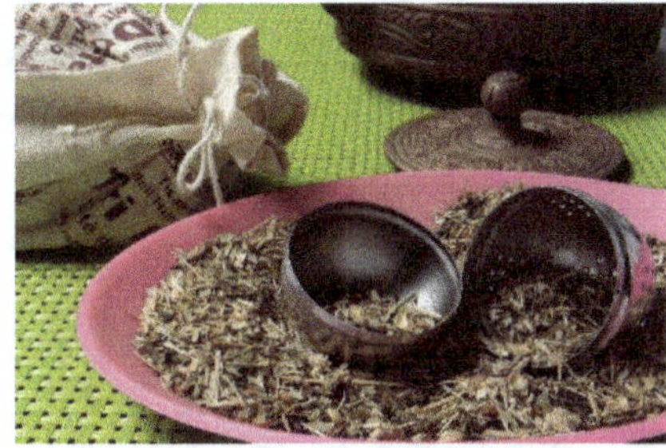

2. **Measure Herbs**: Use about one teaspoon of dried herbs or two teaspoons of fresh herbs per cup of water. Adjust according to taste and the strength of the herb.

3. **Steep**: Pour hot water over the herbs and let them steep for 5-10 minutes. Covering the pot or cup while steeping helps trap the essential oils and flavors.

4. **Strain and Serve**: Strain the tea to remove the herb particles. Serve hot. Sweeteners or lemon may be added according to taste.

16.3 Sample Recipes

- **Peppermint Tea**: Helps soothe digestive ailments.

- o Steep 1-2 teaspoons of dried peppermint leaves in one cup of boiling water for 5-7 minutes.

- **Chamomile Tea**: Aids in relaxation and sleep.

  - o Steep 1-2 teaspoons of dried chamomile flowers in one cup of boiling water for 5-7 minutes.

Chapter 17: Tinctures

Herbal tinctures are concentrated herbal extracts made using alcohol or glycerin. They provide a convenient and effective way to administer herbs, as they preserve the active ingredients for a long period.

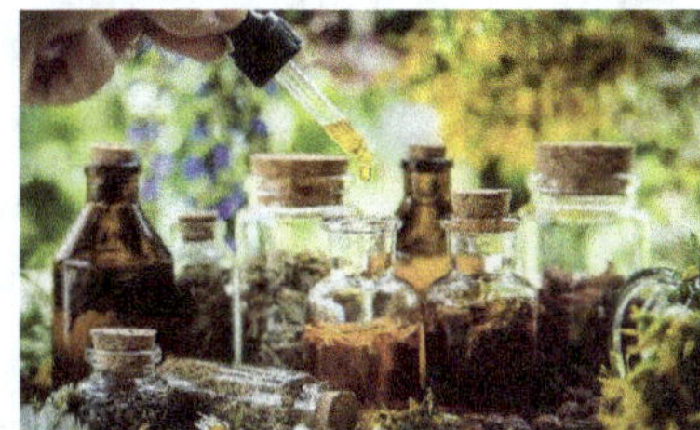

17.1 Making Herbal Tinctures

- **Ingredients**: Fresh or dried herbs, high-proof alcohol (e.g., vodka, brandy) or vegetable glycerin

- **Tools**: Glass jar, strainer, dark dropper bottles

17.2 Steps to Make Tinctures

1. **Prepare Herbs**: Chop fresh herbs or crush dried herbs to increase the surface area for better extraction.

2. **Fill Jar**: Fill a glass jar 1/3 to 1/2 full with herbs. Do not pack tightly.

3. **Add Solvent**: Pour alcohol or glycerin over the herbs until the jar is nearly full. Ensure the herbs are completely submerged to prevent mold growth.

4. **Seal and Store**: Close the jar tightly and store it in a cool, dark place. Let the mixture sit for 4-6 weeks, shaking the jar daily to mix the herbs with the solvent.

5. **Strain**: After the infusion period, strain the tincture through a fine mesh strainer or cheesecloth into another container. Press or squeeze the herbs to extract as much liquid as possible.

6. **Bottle**: Transfer the strained liquid into dark dropper bottles for easy use and storage. Label the bottles with the herb name and date.

17.3 Sample Recipes

- **Milk Thistle Tincture**: Supports liver health.

    o Use 1 part dried milk thistle seeds to 5 parts alcohol. Follow the steps above.

- **Nettle Tincture**: Rich in nutrients and helps with allergies.

- o Use 1 part dried nettle leaves to 5 parts alcohol. Follow the same tincture-making process.

Conclusion

As we conclude "Nature's Cure: A Forager's Guide to Herbal Remedies," we've explored a wide array of herbs, each with unique properties and benefits that can enhance our health and well-being. From the liver-cleansing power of milk thistle to the calming effects of chamomile and the respiratory relief offered by peppermint, these herbs provide accessible, effective, and natural alternatives to many conventional medicines.

Throughout this guide, we have delved into the scientific and traditional backgrounds of these plants, detailing how they can be identified, harvested, and utilized for their medicinal properties. We've seen how milk thistle supports liver health, how dandelion root aids digestion, and how nettles serve as a nutrient powerhouse. Each chapter has aimed to not only educate but also to inspire safer and more informed interactions with the natural world.

We've also discussed the importance of sustainable foraging practices to ensure that these herbal resources remain abundant and continue to thrive in their natural habitats. Conservation efforts are vital for maintaining the balance of our ecosystems and ensuring that future generations can also benefit from these natural remedies.

In addition to individual herb profiles, we've provided practical advice on preparing herbal remedies at home, from tinctures and teas to salves and poultices. This hands-on approach empowers readers to take control of their health in a proactive, informed, and natural way.

Moreover, the bonus chapter on topical applications highlights how herbs can be used for skin health, demonstrating the versatility of herbal medicine not just for internal ailments but also for external healing and care.

As we integrate these herbs into our daily lives, we encourage continued education and consultation with healthcare professionals, especially when integrating herbal remedies with conventional treatments. While herbs offer incredible health benefits, they are most effective when used knowledgeably and respectfully.

This guide has laid the foundation for a journey into herbal medicine, providing the tools and knowledge necessary to explore the healing power of plants. Whether you are a novice forager or an experienced herbalist, "Nature's Cure" offers insights that can enrich your understanding of herbal remedies and enhance your overall health and wellness.

References

1. Di Napoli, A., & Zucchetti, P. (2021). A comprehensive review of the benefits of Taraxacum officinale on human health. BULLETIN OF THE NATIONAL RESEARCH CENTRE, 45(110). https://doi.org/10.1186/s42269-021-00567-1

2. Karimi, G., et al. (2021). Efficacy of Plantago major seed in management of ulcerative colitis symptoms: A randomized, placebo-controlled, clinical trial. COMPLEMENTARY THERAPIES IN CLINICAL PRACTICE, 44, 101444. https://doi.org/10.1016/j.ctcp.2021.101444

3. Jazayeri, S. F., et al. (2021). The Efficacy of Plantago major Seed on Liver Enzymes in Nonalcoholic Fatty Liver Disease: A Randomized Double-Blind Clinical Trial. EVIDENCE-BASED COMPLEMENTARY AND ALTERNATIVE MEDICINE, 2021,

Article ID 6693887. https://doi.org/10.1155/2021/6693887

4. Abidet, A., Gherraf, N., Kalla, A., Zellagui, A., & Fella, O. (2020). Assessment of total phenolics and flavonoids, and evaluation of scavenging activity of the aerial parts of Verbascum thapsus L. and Lactuca virosa L. grown in Algeria. INTERNATIONAL JOURNAL OF CHEMICAL AND BIOCHEMICAL SCIENCES, 17, 86-92.

5. Villalva, M., et al. (2022). Antioxidant, Anti-Inflammatory, and Antibacterial Properties of an Achillea millefolium L. Extract. ANTIOXIDANTS, 11, 1849. https://doi.org/10.3390/antiox11101849

6. Yakhkeshi, S., et al. (2012). Effects of Yarrow on Immune Response and Serum Lipids in Broilers. JOURNAL OF AGRICULTURAL SCIENCE AND TECHNOLOGY, 14, 799-810.

7. Kennedy, D. O. et al. (2003). Modulation of Mood and Cognitive Performance Following Acute Administration of Melissa Officinalis. NEUROPSYCHOPHARMACOLOGY, 28, 1871–1881.

8. Virchea, L.-I. et al. (2021). Phytochemical Analysis and Antioxidant Assay of Melissa Officinalis L. BIO WEB OF CONFERENCES, 40.

9. Ullah, M. A. et al. (2022). Medicinal Benefits of Lemon Balm (Melissa officinalis) for Human Health. WORLD JOURNAL OF CHEMICAL AND PHARMACEUTICAL SCIENCES, 01(01), 028–033.

10. Shabbir, A. et al. (2020). Peppermint Oil, Its Useful, and Adverse Effects on Human Health: A Review. INNOVARE JOURNAL OF AYURVEDIC SCIENCE.

11. Chakraborty, A. et al. (2022). Bioactive components of peppermint (Mentha piperita L.), their pharmacological and ameliorative potential and ethnomedicinal benefits: A review. JOURNAL OF PHARMACOGNOSY AND PHYTOCHEMISTRY.

12. Wieland, L.S., et al. (2021). Elderberry for prevention and treatment of viral respiratory illnesses: a systematic review. BMC COMPLEMENTARY MEDICINE AND THERAPIES, 21(112). https://doi.org/10.1186/s12906-021-03283-5

13. Charlebois, D. (2007). Elderberry as a medicinal plant. In ISSUES IN NEW CROPS AND NEW USES (pp. 284-292). ASHS Press, Alexandria, VA.

About Our Team

Value Guides is a small, closeknit publishing organization with a variety of professionals either in-house or to whom we contract assignments. We strive to relay our enthusiasm for knowledge in a succinct way for our busy readers.

9 798324 864613